THE STRESS AND ANXIETY MEDKIT

Felicity karon.

©2023 Felicity Karon

Introduction

Stress is the sensation of being beneath an excessive amount of intellectual or emotional stress.Pressure will become stress when you are unable to handle your situation. People have one-of-a-kind approaches of reacting to stress, so a situation that feels traumatic to someone can be motivating to another person.

Stress isn't an ailment itself, but it can lead to extreme illness if it isn't attended to in due time. It's important to recognise the symptoms of pressure early. Recognising the symptoms and signs of stress will help you discern out approaches of coping and help you not to adopt bad coping strategies, like taking excessive liquor or smoking. Take note that there's no cure to stress, it can only be managed.

Chapter 1

<u>Meaning of stress</u>

Stress is a feeling of emotional or physical tension. It can come from any event or notion that makes you to become annoyed, indignant, or frightened. Stress is your body's reaction to a venture or demand. In brief bursts, stress can be good, which include why it aids you keep away from danger or meet a deadline. But when stress lasts for a long term, it is able to damage your health.

Stress can be defined as any type of adjustment that causes physical, emotional or psychological pressure. Stress is your body's reaction to whatever that requires interest or motion. Everyone stories strain to a few diploma. The way you respond to stress, however, makes a large difference on your standard well-being.

Stress can purpose or influence the direction of many scientific situations including mental situations along with depression and anxiety. Medical issues that result from stress, include poor recuperation, irritable bowel syndrome, excessive blood strain, poorly managed diabetes and plenty of other conditions. Stress management is recognized as an powerful treatment modality to encompass pharmacologic and non-pharmacologic components.

In medical term, the body's response to bodily, intellectual, or emotional pressure. Stress causes chemical changes inside the body that could improve blood stress, coronary heart pumping, and blood sugar ranges. It might also result in emotions of frustration, anxiety, anger, or melancholy. Stress may be resulting from everyday lifestyles activities or by means of an event, inclusive of trauma or infection. Long-term strain or excessive levels of strain can also cause mental and bodily health problems.

Anxiety on the other hand, is an emotion characterised with the aid of feelings of tension, worried thoughts, and physical modifications like improved blood strain.

People with anxiety issues generally have recurring intrusive mind or concerns. They may also keep away from certain situations out of fear. They might also have physical symptoms including perspiring, trembling, dizziness, or a rapid heartbeat.

 Anxiety is a complicated response to real or perceived threats. It can involve cognitive, physical, and behavioral changes.

Real or perceived risk reasons a rush of adrenaline, a

hormone and chemical messenger in the brain, which in turn triggers these anxiety reactions in a technique known as the combat-or-flight reaction. Some people may additionally enjoy this reaction in hard social situations or around important activities or decisions.

The period or severity of emotions of anxiety can occasionally be out of share to the authentic trigger or stressor. Physical signs, which includes multiplied blood stress and nausea, may also develop. These responses flow past tension into an tension ailment.

Once anxiety reaches the stage of a sickness, it can interfere with daily characteristic. In a lame man's term, the difference between stress and anxiety is that, the former is due to an existing strain-inflicting thing or "stressor", while the latter is the stressor that maintains after the stressor is gone. So it is able to be conferred that tension is the after math of pressure

Stress is a regular feeling. There are predominant varieties of stress:

Acute stress: This is brief-time period stress that is going away fast. You sense it when you slam at the brakes, have a fight with your partner, or ski down a steep slope. It helps you manipulate risky situations. It also happens when you do something new or thrilling.

All humans have acute stress at one time or any other.

Chronic stress: This is stress that lasts for an extended time period. You may additionally have continual stress if you have money issues, an unhappy marriage, or trouble at work. Any form of pressure that is going on for weeks or months is chronic pressure. You can grow to be so used to persistent pressure which you do not recognise it's miles a trouble. If you do not find ways to manage stress, it is able to lead to fitness issues.

Chapter 2

<u>Common causes of stress</u>

Stress is an everyday thing and, to a degree, an essential part of lifestyles. Despite it being some thing all people experience, what reasons stress can vary from person to individual.

For example, one man or woman may also come to be irritated and beaten via a serious traffic jam, even as any other might turn up their music and take it into account as a moderate inconveniences.

What's causing you strain may already be something you are abundantly privy to. But given the importance of maintaining stress in check with regards to mitigating the results it is able to have in your bodily and intellectual health, it is well worth commencing yourself to know that other elements can be at play, too. Craft your stress-discount plan with they all in mind.

❖ Financial Problems:

Money concerns are one of the essential sources of stress, and might lead to relationship troubles, depression or anxiety.

Some signs that monetary pressure is affecting your health and relationships include arguing with the humans closest to you about money, feeling angry or apprehensive, mood swings, tiredness, muscle ache, lack of appetite, decrease sex pressure and withdrawing from others.

While those are everyday reactions, they could have an effect on your health if they retain for a variety of weeks. You may be susceptible to developing anxiety or despair. Some human beings use drugs or alcohol to help them cope. Some have mind of self-harm or suicide.

People from all walks of life enjoy troubles with cash. It's essential now not to keep it all to yourself and try to deal with it alone.

Signs of financial stress might also encompass:

Arguing with loved ones, being afraid to open mail or solution the telephone, feeling responsible about spending cash on non-essentials, worrying and feeling stressful about cash, etc.

In the lengthy-time period, stress associated with financial issues results in distress, which can also carry up blood stress and reason headaches, disenchanted stomach, chest ache, insomnia, and a well known feeling of sickness. Financial stress has also been linked to a number of health problems, which includes depression, anxiety, skin troubles, diabetes, and arthritis.

❖ Work:

Any variety of things can make contributions to process stress, inclusive of too much work, activity lack of confidence, dissatisfaction with a job or profession, and conflicts with a managing director and/or co-employees.

Whether you're worried about a particular venture or feeling unfairly handled, putting your task ahead of the whole thing else can affect many elements of your life, which includes personal relationships and intellectual and physical health.

Factors outdoor of the process itself actually have a position in paintings stress, consisting of someone's mental makeup, preferred health, personal existence. And the amount of emotional assist they have outside of work.

The signs of work-associated strain can be physical and psychological, such as:

Anxiety,Depression,Difficulty concentrating or making selections, Fatigue,Headache,Heart palpitations,Mood swings,Muscle tension and ache and Stomach problems.

❖ Personal Relationships:

There are humans in all of our lives that cause us stress. It may be a family member, an intimate associate, friend, or co-worker. Toxic people lurk in all elements of our lives and the stress we revel in from those relationships can have an effect on physical and intellectual health.

There are several causes of stress in romantic relationships and while couples are continuously underneath stress, the relationship can be at the danger of failure.

Common courting stressors include:

1. Being too busy to spend time with each other and percentage responsibilities,

2. Intimacy and sex end up rare due to commercial enterprise, health problems, and any wide variety of different reasons

3. There is abuse or control within the relationship

4. You and your accomplice are not speaking

5. You and/or associate are ingesting too much alcohol and/or using tablets

6. You or your companion are thinking about divorce

7. The signs of stress associated with non-public relationships are much like regular signs and symptoms of trendy pressure and can consist of bodily health and sleep problems, depression, and anxiety.

You might also locate yourself avoiding or having struggle with the character, or becoming effortlessly indignant by using their presence.

Sometimes, personal dating stress also can be associated with our relationships with people on social media platforms, such as Facebook. For example, social media tends to certainly encourage evaluating yourself to others, which could cause the stress of feeling insufficient. It additionally makes bullying simpler.

❖   Parenting:

Parents are frequently faced with dealing with busy schedules that include a process, family responsibilities, and raising kids. These demands bring about parenting stress.

High stages of parenting stress can cause a mother or father to be harsh, negative, and authoritarian in their interactions with their kids. Parenting stress can also decrease the excellent of parent-child relationships. For instance, you could not have open communication so your child doesn't come to you for recommendation otherwise you and your baby may also argue often.

Sources of parenting strain may additionally consist of being decrease-earnings, working long hours, single parenting, marital or relationship tensions, or elevating a baby who has been recognized with a behavioral ailment or developmental incapacity.

Parents of kids with behavior disorders and developmental delays have the very best risk for parenting stress. In truth, several studies display mother and father of children with autistic characteristics are reporting better tiers of parenting stress than human beings whose children do not have the condition.

❖ Daily Life and Busyness:

Day-to-day stressors are our every day inconveniences. They include such things as misplacing keys, going for walks overdue, and forgetting to convey an important object with you when leaving the house. Usually, these are simply minor setbacks, but in the event that they emerge as common, they grow to be a supply of hysteria affecting bodily and/or psychological fitness.

The pressure of being too busy is getting an increasing number of common. These days, people are busier than ever and that provides plenty of strain to their lives.

In some cases, busyness is due to necessity, together with having to work a 2nd job. Other times, it is because of guilt and not looking to disappoint others. People won't say "no" and turn out to be having little time for themselves, or they forget about their personal primary needs, which include consuming right and exercise because of lack of time.

❖   Personality and Resources:

Your personal traits and the assets you have got available to you tie into all of the above and can be independent sources of stress as well.

Extroverts, as an instance, tend to experience much less stress in every day lifestyles and feature greater social sources, which buffer against pressure. Perfectionists, however, can also carry stress onto themselves unnecessarily due to their exacting requirements, experiencing more terrible mental and physical fitness outcomes than folks who merely focus on high achievement.

Those who're "type A" can pressure absolutely everyone round them, consisting of themselves. Those with sufficient money to rent help can delegate demanding responsibilities, so this resource can offer an area over folks who war to make ends meet and must paintings more difficult to save coins.

Chapter 3

<u>Adverse effects of stress</u>

One very popular effect of stress is depression. Emotional stress can play a position in inflicting melancholy(depression) or be a symptom of it. An annoying state of affairs can trigger feelings of despair, and those emotions could make it extra difficult to cope with stress.

High-stress occasions, inclusive of losing a job or the breaking up of a serious courtship, can lead to depression. Not every body who experiences those situations turns into depressed, others may end up with other physical disorders.

Stress has affected people in a harmful manner for the duration of time. It is recognized when the man or woman passes through a sure tragedy or uncomfortable moment of their life, the body can routinely discover if the state of affairs the character is going through is both threatening or non-threatening to them, and stress can both have an effect on them long time or for a short quantity of time. Stress factors also rely on the man or woman's gender, age, character, etc.

The individuals will react in exclusive methods, a few may also react very irritating, coronary heart beat goes quicker, their blood pressure rises, breathing is a lot heavier, the muscle mass tighten up. This helps the character to react quicker to a scenario, as an instance, when you are approximately to have a automobile accident, your body reacts to access the car's break that allows you to prevent any damage.

The human body is designed to react to stress, for you to shield itself in opposition to threats or any aggressive conditions or individual, that portrays a hazard to oneself. Stressors, as an instance, can be and are job-associated situations, being disturbed too much about presenting for his or her own family, while looking after family contributors which includes children or elderly spouse and children, that require greater assist and extra care. In which the body mechanically considers a stressor as a hazard.

Stressors are constantly found in our existence due to living in a very fast-paced society, in which every body demands to do everything efficiently and in a sure amount of quick time. The body can automatically feel insecure, and the fight-or-flight response may occur.

Stressful existence occasions come before tension or anxiety disorders. Negative affects of Stress in an man or woman existence will possibly motive health terrible impacts after stressful occasions in their life. Many human beings suppose that being tipsy, smoking, using any type of substance, or maybe napping more than usual, the use of the net, or seeing movies might also assist them, and relax them for the moment, but in reality, their depression or any other disease may additionally worsen.

Stress significantly damages the nicely-being of someone. It makes each day life hard and damages intimate relationships, and feature a harmful impact on human health. When a person is below colossal Stress, they behave as a result. It from time to time, takes an emotional toll on humans, and a light diploma of Stress may also generate frustrations and slight tension, however prolonged Stress should generate despair, anxiety sickness, and burnout.

Constant stress at the body has critical bodily fitness outcomes. Some of the poor bodily outcomes of chronic stress are due to the extreme pressure reaction, which hampers digestion, will increase blood pumping, makes the heart beat quicker, and floods your body with extra chemicals. This makes the coronary heart work a whole lot harder than it desires to, and it's not wholesome to be in a constant, worked-up condition. That is why one of the predominant long-term fitness results of stress is cardiovascular ailment, such as heart sickness, excessive blood pressure, coronary heart assaults, and stroke. Other physical consequences of continual stress may be because of the manner humans cope with stress. For example, eating unbalanced diet with too much carbohydrates, coupled with a loss of exercise can lead to obesity. Chronic pressure can appreciably impair someone's physical health.

Mental fitness issues also are many of the primary poor outcomes of chronic pressure. Depression and anxiety are very common in folks that continuously file excessive stages of stress. Many research have shown that this connection is more than truly a correlation. These intellectual fitness outcomes are sincerely a result of the pressure many humans experience.

In addition to health, pressure can negatively affect human behavior. The stress reaction also has a position to play here. When the body reacts to stress, blood is pulled from the prefrontal cortex and goes to the emotion centers of our mind. This influences the logical processes of the human mind. Without enough blood flowing to the logical center of the brain, humans often lack intellectual readability or the ability to make choices nicely. As a result, people who suffer from persistent pressure may not appear to make the pleasant decision in life. They may also rush right into a selection or have a tough time prioritizing what desires to be executed. Many at times, they do not completely take into account the implications of an action the equal way that they might have in the event that they weren't underneath a lot stress.

By and large, stress has natural repercussions and can have lasting effects. Stress can come because of jobs or changes in existence and it could lead to considerable fitness issues and adjustments in behavior. Because stress is so common for people living in our fast-paced lives, we have to understand the realities of stress before we take steps to try to alternate it. Remember that stress isn't terrible; but it's prolonged exposure to stressors without a smash that without a doubt does the harm. Once the realities are understood, we have to take steps to govern our very own pressure stages so we are able to live and enjoy a long, healthy and happier lifestyles.

Chapter 4

<u>Meditation as a way of controlling stress</u>

Meditation has many benefits, which includes reducing stress, improving immune characteristic, and slowing intellectual ageing. This age-old practice has come to be one of the most popular ways to alleviate pressure among humans of all walks of life. Meditation can take many paperwork and may be mixed with many religious practices. It also can be used in several important approaches.

It can be a part of your daily routine and assist you build resilience to stress.

It can be a technique to get targeted while you're thrown off through emotional pressure.

It may be a quick-repair pressure reliever to help you change your body's stress reaction and physically loosen up.

Your bodily and emotional stress can soften away by way of getting to know to calm your body and mind. This leaves you feeling higher, refreshed, and geared up to face the challenges of your day with a wholesome mindset. With everyday practice over weeks or months, you could experience even more blessings.

What is Meditation?

Meditation is a practice that includes exclusive strategies that assist human beings remove their attention from lots of things and obtain a high state of consciousness. It can bring about adjustments in consciousness and has been shown to have some of health advantages.

Meditation involves sitting in a relaxed function and clearing your mind, or focusing your thoughts on one notion and clearing it of all others.

A well known thread most of the many meditation techniques is that the thoughts stops following each new idea that involves the floor.

It's commonly important to have as a maximum of half an hour free from distractions, although meditation sessions can truly be any length. Longer meditation sessions have a tendency to bring extra advantages, but it is usually best to start slowly so you can hold the exercise long-term.

Many humans discover that if they try to meditate for too long every session or create a "ideal" exercise it is able to grow to be intimidating or daunting, and they see it as extra challenging to maintain as a daily routine. It is best to create the routine and do it into a more thorough way of that addiction.

It's useful to have silence and privacy, however more experienced meditators can practice meditation everywhere.

Many people who engage in meditations attach a spiritual component to it, however it may also be a mundane exercise. Really, there's no wrong way to meditate.

One of the main advantages of meditation is its potential to lessen stress. The body's stress reaction causes it to routinely react in approaches that put together you to fight or run. In a few cases of extreme chance, this bodily response is beneficial. However, a prolonged condition of such agitation can be a repercussion to physical damage to every part of the body.

Meditation impacts the body in precisely the alternative way that stress does—with the aid of awakening the body's relaxation response. It revives the body to a relaxed condition, assisting the body to restore itself and preventing new damage from the physical consequences of stress.

A greater advantage that meditation can deliver is the long-term strength that can come with ordinary exercise.

Research has proven that people who practice meditation frequently begin to experience adjustments of their response to stress that allow them to recover from worrying situations more easily and revel in much less pressure from the demanding situations they face of their ordinary lives.

During meditation, you centre your attention and quiet the movement of jumbled mind that can be crowding your thoughts and causing stress. Meditation can instill a feel of calm, peace and stability that could put your emotional health and your basic fitness at a great advantage The practice of getting to know how refocus your thoughts also can assist you redirect yourself while you fall into negative questioning patterns, which in itself can help relieve stress. Meditation offers several answers in one simple hobby.

The blessings of meditation are superb because, amongst other things, it is able to change your stress reaction, thereby protecting you from the consequences of chronic stress.

When working towards meditation:

- ❖ You breath more successfully.

- ❖ Your adrenal glands produce less cortisol.

- ❖ Your blood stress normalizes.

- ❖ Your coronary heart charge and respiration gradual down.

- ❖ Your immune system is boosted.

- ❖ Your thoughts ages at a slower price.

- ❖ Your mind is freed and your rate of creativity increases

- ❖ You perspire much less.

People who meditate often find it less difficult to surrender life-detrimental behavior like smoking, ingesting, and abuse of drugs.

Chapter 5

<u>Rest and sleep as another control of stress</u>

Sleep is a powerful pressure and stress reducer. Following a normal sleep pattern calms and restores the system, improves concentration, regulates mood, and sharpens judgment and decision-making. You are a higher hassle solver and are higher able to cope with stress when you're well-rested. Lack of sleep, on the other hand, reduces your strength and diminishes mental clarity.

High-pleasant sleep can have a extremely fine effect on our health, consisting of a reduced threat of heart disease, stroke, and diabetes. It may even increase your mood and cleanse your skin. One of the most impactful advantages, however, is the impact it is able to have on stress ranges.

While some stress is natural, an excessive amount of it is able to be destructive for your health. Some pressure may be because of specific internal and environmental factors, but it is basically impacted with the aid of how much sleep you get, or don't get. With a growing variety of over-worked adults, getting enough sleep has emerge as a more and more essential and healthful way of life choice.

Sleep's potential to alter the immune system, or even enhance it, is a critical thing of a stress-loose lifestyles. We all understand sickness isn't fun, but it also adds plenty of problems to an already busy body. Along with intellectual stress, sickness in one part of the body puts quite a few bodily stress on the relaxation of your systems, inflicting them to overwork and strain themselves to exertion.

While you sleep, however, your body takes charge over itself and produces materials that fight and guard against any ailment and infection. Therefore, getting the sleep you want to keep your immune system can enhance your reaction to infection, shorten the time it takes to get better, and allow you to get back to everyday existence.

Losing an excessive amount of sleep can spark off an area of the mind that controls emotional processing and worry. While people with an anxiety ailment are much more likely to experience the mental results of a lack of sleep, it may nonetheless impact anybody who doesn't get sufficient rest. It can overwork the coronary heart and become the cause of severe stress, negatively affecting your mental fitness and how you deal with social situations. Not getting enough sleep can lead to a terrible mood, low strength, difficulty concentrating, and a widespread incapacity to function as expected. Lack of sleep can also have severe consequences in a few instances, such as if someone is driving or running heavy equipment while worn-out. The occasional night of negative sleep is not likely to cause harm, however persistent sleep deprivation can increase the chance of several persistent fitness conditions.

Adequate sleep, however, has been verified to significantly lessen emotions of tension by way of enhancing your capacity to react to stress in the best manner. Specifically, an amazing night time's sleep can increase your mood, outlook and temperament.

You may discover that you can't pay attention as effortlessly with out sleep. I

Loss of sleep renders you extra emotionally reactive,

extra impulsive, and greater touchy to negative stimuli. These sleep-driven cognitive impairments can provide rise to stress in any wide variety of ways, from developing issue in relationships to inflicting issues with job overall performance.

There are many strategies that can help you control strain in order that it doesn't intrude with sleep. Taking time to relax and wind down before going to bed is important to having a good night rest and doing away with the pressure of the day. A period of quiet time before bed time permits you to step faraway from every day worries and set them apart before you go to bed. Try taking a warm bathe or bath, getting a rubdown or doing a little light stretching before bed.Set your bedtime and stick to it – An often sleep schedule of going to sleep and waking up at the same time every day, even on weekends. It may be a challenge before everything, however give it time—as your body system adjusts, you'll in all likelihood find that a regular bedtime feels right.

Although the affects of tension issues may be enormous, they may be one of the maximum treatable mental health issues. This doesn't mean that lowering tension is always easy, however there are treatments which could help.

Any individual who has chronic or enormous anxiety and/or sound asleep issues ought to talk with a medical doctor who can fine check their situation and talk the pros and cons of the remedy options in their case.Both your sleep conduct and environment are part of sleep hygiene. Steps to improve sleep hygiene encompass making your bed extra comfy, eliminating sources of sleep disruption like light and noise, and keeping off caffeine and alcohol in the afternoon and evening.

Trying rest techniques can help pick out ways to dispose of anxiety and make it less complicated to fall asleep quick and peacefully. Relaxation exercises can destroy the cycle of fear and rumination. You can also want to try scheduling instances to actively fear worry about things that bother you, as this can get rid of annoying time as you lay down for sleep. Deep respiration, mindfulness meditation, and guided imagery are only some tactics to relaxation that could assist in placing your thoughts at-ease before bedtime or if you awaken at some point of the night.

Chapter 6

Exercise and balance diet as a control of stress

In reality, there is little or nothing you could do about the pressure in your life. What you could do something about, but, is how you allow it affect you. And the great vicinity to start is with a bedrock of healthy living. This solid foundation may also help guard you against the dangerous consequences of the chronic stress all of us live with.That means following a healthy lifestyle, specifically with regards to feeding and keeping fit.

Eating balanced diet can support a healthy immune system and the repair of broken cells. It gives the extra strength needed to address worrying occasions. If you regularly rely on fast foods because you are tired or too busy to prepare food at your place of residence , think about meal making plans, a practice which could help manage time in the end, make certain balanced healthy food, and prevent weight gain.

When we eat under stress, we devour quickly without noticing what or how lots we're consuming, that could cause weight gain. Mindful ingesting practices counteract pressure by encouraging deep breaths, making considerate food picks, focusing attention at the meal, and chewing meals slowly and carefully. This increases enjoyment of the meal and improves digestion.

Eating a wholesome diet can reduce the bad effects of stress to your body, a healthy food plan builds a strong, extra enduring immunity in your body with the aid of lowering oxidation and inflammation and through helping to lessen weight benefit."

Healthy dieting is not simple to keep up, especially when you're always busy and stressed. For many, prepping wholesome meals doesn't continually fit into a hectic agenda and eating out is the norm at times.

This usually contributes to a much less healthy diet, all of us know how easy it's far to treat ourselves to that wealthy, high-fat meal we have been craving — but might usually not repair for ourselves."

For this reason, building a healthy food prep addiction into your each day or weekly routine can substantially enhance your average weight loss plan, and in the end lead to decreased stress rates.

Eating at home usually will increase the chance that you'll consume a wholesome diet, one way to make it easier to devour a wholesome eating diet is to keep clean nutritious foods in stock. Many also can be stored frozen or dried — like nuts and high fiber cereals. A balanced and wholesome weight-reduction plan is prior to supporting our bodies to manage the physiological changes resulting from stress. A critical part of any pressure reaction consists of figuring out and reducing the causes of stress. Skip the easy sugars and starches. The spike in blood sugar and insulin, combined with your already excessive sugar degrees, can lead you to consume extra in addition to placing you prone to insulin insensitivity and diabetes. There's nothing incorrect with reaching for consolation meals, however take the attributes of the "bad" consolation meals - creamy, crunchy, sweet - and try and find healthier alternatives.

Avoid coffee and different caffeinated food and drink. They no longer handiest increase degrees of certain stress hormones, however additionally mimic their effects in the body (increasing heart beat, as an example).

Load up on greens and fruits and other excessive-fiber meals. The vitamins they offer lend a further dollop of protection towards the immune-sapping results of continual pressure.

Exercise in almost any shape can act as a stress reliever.

You realize that exercise does your body well, but you are too busy and stressed to match it into your schedule. In relation to exercise and pressure, the good news is that virtually any form of exercise, from aerobics to yoga, can act as a stress reliever. If you're no longer an athlete or maybe if you're out of shape, you can still make a touch exercising move a protracted way towards stress management.

Exercise will increase your general fitness and your sense of properly-being, which puts extra liveliness in your doorstep every day. But exercise also has a few direct pressure-busting advantages.

It reduces bad consequences of stress. Exercise can provide pressure comfort to your body at the same time as imitating effects of stress, inclusive of the flight or fight reaction, and assisting your body and its structures work together to eliminate worries. This can

also result in fine consequences for your body —
inclusive of your cardiovascular, digestive and immune
systems — by aiding guard your body from dangerous
results of stress.

It's meditation in motion. After a quick-paced game of
racquetball, a long walk or run, or numerous laps within
the pool, you can regularly discover which you've
forgotten the day's irritations and concentrated only in
your body's actions.

As you start to regularly shed your daily tensions
through motion and physical activity, you may discover
that placing your mind in the activity only, and the
ensuing strength and positivity, allow you to stay calm,
clean and focused in the whole lot you do.

It improves your mood. Regular exercise can elevate
your self-esteem, improve your temper, assist you
loosen up, and lower signs and symptoms of moderate
melancholy and tension. Exercise also can improve
your sleep, that's often disturbed by stress, depression
and anxiety. All of those exercise benefits can ease
your stress rates and offer you a sense of command
over your body and your lifestyles.

When you've been diagnosed with heart ailment, you want to manage a variety of of recent stressors on an ongoing basis. Dealing with more common medical doctor visits, getting used to new clinical treatments, and adjusting to lifestyle changes are just some of the elements that can reason you to experience stress and anxiety.

Fortunately, you can take some easy steps to assist relieve stress. Many of these steps can help improve your basic health as well, including your heart's health. Exercise is one of the exceptional strategies for fighting stress and handling heart sickness.

Physical hobby can help lower your general stress tiers and enhance your quality of life, either mentally and physically. Exercising regularly can have a nice impact on your temper through relieving the tension, anger, and mild melancholy that frequently move hand-in-hand with stress. It can enhance the high-quality of your sleep, which may be negatively impacted with the aid of stress, melancholy, and anxiety. It also can assist enhance your self esteem.

Physical activity improves your body's potential to use

oxygen and also improves blood movement round the body. Both of these changes have a positive effect on your brain. This is the sense of feeling good and euphoria that many humans experience after exercising. Physical engagements can also help take your thoughts off your issues. The repetitive movements in exercising leads you to place your attention on your body, rather than your mind. By concentrating at the rhythm of your movements, you experience some of the advantages of meditation while doing the exercise. Focusing on a sole physical mission can produce a experience of strength and positivity. This a centre can help offer peace and clarity.

Some humans noted an improvement of their mood immediately after a exercise. Those feelings don't cease there, however typically come to be cumulative over time. Chances are, you'll discover accelerated feelings of properly-being as you stay committed to a consistent workout schedule.

In addition to having a direct impact on your stress rates, doing workout often also promotes most fulfilling fitness in other methods. Improvements to your normal fitness may additionally help accidentally moderate your stress rates. So, in improving your diet and body fitness, you'll hardly feel stressed at the long-run.

Chapter 7

<u>Music as a mind healer</u>

Music has long been acknowledged to be a strong stress reliever. In reality, music is one of the most commonly used equipment for stress alleviation. There are many different methods that music may be used for anxiety remedy.Some human beings find that listening to calm, relaxing tune aids in diminishing their pressure level. Others might also prefer to pay attention to track with a quicker tempo so that it will assist worries get out of their head and into the tune.

Music may have a profound effect on both the feelings and the body. Faster song can make your sense extra alert and concentrate higher. Upbeat tune can make you feel extra constructive and fantastic approximately life. A slower pace can quiet your mind and relax your muscles, making you feel soothed at the same time as releasing the pressure of the day. Music is powerful for relaxation and stress control.

Listening to track is influential. It can set the temper in sure conditions, deliver past nostalgic memories, and in a few instances, even assist relieve stress.

In fact, the energy of music for stress comfort may be

extremely good. As it influences us with its relaxing outcomes on our minds and our bodies, in turn, it also allows to alleviate pressure. This approach taking note of music just is probably the solution for individuals who are trying to soften their stresses away.

Stress may be reduced and relaxation maximized with the use of song, specially when it's a classical song. This gradual and quiet genre has an effect on physiological functions because the pulse and heart beat are slowed down.Blood strain also can be reduced along with pressure hormones whilst listening to classical track. This paves way for a calm experience and a excellent way to manipulate the worries that always lingers in your mind.Music is also known to have a deep effect on our feelings. Slower tempos can assist to silence the mind and loosen up muscle tissue, making song a powerful stress control device.

Sometimes you need something to take your thoughts off of your stresses. Music can be a high-quality tool for supplying distractions because it absorbs interest and diverts focus.Music can be a remarkable addition to meditation because it allows to maintain the mind from wandering and helps to offer rest. The preference of song could be extraordinary for anyone, as everyone is particular in how track influences them. It may also depend on the mood we're in at the time.Music might even be a helpful distraction to people who are stressful or are experiencing pain. Distractions can be amazing for taking the thoughts off of more difficult conditions and making you feel plenty better at some point of them.

Now, speaking contrary to music as a distraction – music also can be a tool for increasing productiveness. The sort of track is in reality what matters on the subject of slowing down or making productivity faster.Faster track can help you to sense more alert and assist to boom productivity. More upbeat tune also can assist you to feel more positive and assist you to better maintain a balanced mind set.

When your pressure levels are high, it might seem natural to try to stay far from taking note of tune in an effort to solve your stresses. But being attentive to song is amazing for lowering stress and increasing productivity, or can at least help in assisting you towards it.You might make song part of your normal schedule to assist calm your stress, with the aid of being attentive to it inside the automobile, while exercising, or at the same time as taking your morning shower. Including music with your day to day activities is a exquisite way to reduce stress or be higher organized for it while it comes your way.

Losing sleep is a not unusual problem for individuals who suffer from stress. Music can help with generating sleep as it is able to have an impact on physical, psychological and emotional states which make contributions to the success of sleep. When you are too alert or excited before bed, it becomes a lot extra tough to move into a drowsy.

Listening to soothing music is an extraordinary manner to help you wind down and relax earlier before you sleep. Sleep high-quality is also boosted as awaken instances during the night time emerge as much less. You will wake up feeling a great deal greater refreshed inside the morning as your body stays calm during the night time.Relaxing song can trigger the discharge of feel-good chemical substances in the brain. Your adventure to sleep is stepped forward as your heart beat is diminished and respiratory bogged down.

If you've ever belted out your favourite tune then you recognize how correct singing alongside to tune can be for the soul. Sometimes it just feels necessary so one can push through a greater tough time.

Singing alongside is a first way to release tension and make your self feel excellent. When you feel proper, you're much more likely to relax and let go of your stress. This then helps you to cope with demanding instances in a more calm and prepared fashion.

One key gain of paying attention to music for pressure management is that it improves your immune system's operation. In addition, music has been discovered to increase the activity of natural killer cells, which might be an essential part of the immune system's protection in opposition to viruses and bacteria. Therefore, incorporating music right into a stress control schedule can't simplest reduce stress in the meanwhile but additionally improve normal health and properly-being.

One method to include music into your every day schedule as a stress management method is to concentrate to peaceful or uplifting tune even as training deep respiratory or meditation. This can help to relax the frame and clear the mind thereby lowering pressure level.

Another concept is to have a delegated time each day for paying attention to music, whether it be throughout a exercise or at the same time as cooking dinner. Music can serve as a distraction from daily duties and responsibilities, offering a much-wanted break from annoying situations. Additionally, paying attention to music also can enhance temper and improve universal emotions of excitement and optimism.You also can use song as a way of active rest through undertaking bodily sports which include yoga or meditation at the same time as listening to calming tunes.

By and large, incorporating music into your daily routine as a stress management tactic can promote rest and emotional well-being. Do not get overwhelmed by your emotions, instead learn to control them. Welcome each day with good thoughts in your mind to have a great day. Always have a sketch of how you want your day to look like and stay positive.

* 9 7 9 8 3 7 7 0 5 8 4 2 7 *